Belly Fat

51 Quick & Simple Habits to Burn Belly Fat & Tone Abs!

by Linda Westwood

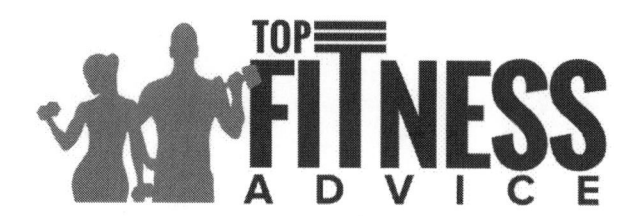

Copyright © 2018 By Linda Westwood
All rights reserved. No part of this book may be reproduced in any form without permission in writing from the author. No part of this publication may be reproduced or transmitted in any form or by any means, mechanic, electronic, photocopying, recording, by any storage or retrieval system, or transmitted by email without the permission in writing from the author and publisher.
For information regarding permissions write to author at Linda@TopFitnessAdvice.com.
Reviewers may quote brief passages in review.

Linda Westwood
TopFitnessAdvice.com

Table of Contents

Who is this book for? _____ 4
What will this book teach you? _____ 5
Introduction _____ 6
Powerful Eating Habits _____ 8
Powerful Workout Habits _____ 69
Powerful Lifestyle Habits _____ 121
Conclusion _____ 143
Final Words _____ 145
Disclaimer _____ 146

Who is this book for?

Are you struggling to lose those last few pounds off your belly?

Are you sick and tired of endless crunches and sit-ups with NO results?

Do you ever wish you could just melt your belly fat *without even trying?*

Then this book is for you!

I am going to share with you some of the MOST effective habits that, when applied, will help YOU burn your belly fat without even trying – because they are going to be habits embedded into your life!

I have put it all together in this comprehensive book containing 51 of the most powerful habits that you can apply for maximum change in minimum time!

Since there is more to burning belly fat than exercise alone, or even diet alone, I have broken this book down into three separate sections for your benefit!

You can be a complete beginner or someone who works out regularly, it doesn't matter!

If this sounds like it could help you, then keep reading…

What will this book teach you?

Inside, I will teach you in great detail how you can start melting your belly fat without too much extra effort!

How? Because you're going to learn which habits are the most powerful and effective at burning belly fat.

Once you learn what these are, and start applying them into your life, you will effortlessly begin seeing your belly trim up and become lean!

In this book, I give you 51 of some of the most powerful and effective belly fat burning habits that you can apply to your life.

One of the most important things for you to realize when reading this book is that the habits *really do work!*

However...

For you to achieve *real success* with these habits, you HAVE to apply them to your life *consistently.*

This is where most people fail – they try out a few habits and then just forget about them all, or even worse, read through the entire book but do nothing.

You MUST try your best to apply these habits as you read through the book!

Introduction

This book will give you the information that you need to start taking control of your health and losing belly fat right now.

If you haven't been able to lose weight before it's not because you don't have enough willpower, it's because you didn't have the right information.

How you eat, how you work out and how you live your life all impact your weight. Once you finish this book you'll know how to make better choices and live a healthier life forever.

Here's what you'll learn:

20 Eating Habits

The food that you eat is fuel for your body. These 20 healthy habits will teach you to eat food that is healthy and tastes good so that you will be able to lose fat and still not feel deprived.

Dieting doesn't help you lose weight, but changing the way that you eat and the way that you think about food will help you lose weight and keep it off forever.

20 Workout Habits

Working out doesn't have to be a chore. Changing your workout habits and finding exercises that you really enjoy will change the way that you view exercise.

Your body was made to move. Working out can be something that you enjoy when you change the way that you exercise to get the most out of your workouts.

Even if you have trouble working out at first you'll find that as you keep going it will get easier because the more you move your body the better your body will move.

11 Lifestyle Habits

Getting healthy means making some lifestyle changes. But, changing your lifestyle doesn't mean that you have to make sweeping or radical changes in order to see positive results.

Small changes in your lifestyle and way of thinking will add up to big results. Changing your lifestyle in healthy ways will not only help you lose weight it will also help you lower your stress level, increase your overall health, and make you happier for the rest of your life.

Give these changes a chance and you will be amazed at how you can transform your body and your life.

Powerful Eating Habits

Changing your relationship with food is the best way to lose fat and stay healthy for the rest of your life.

Do you know why diets don't work?

Diets don't work because they don't change the way that you view food. In order to lose weight and keep it off you need to change your entire approach to eating instead of just restricting what you eat.

You don't need to deprive yourself of food in order to lose weight or stay at a healthy weight. You need to eat the foods that will nourish and sustain your body instead of eating food that will hurt your body.

And don't be fooled into thinking that what you're eating isn't hurting your body.

Obesity numbers are at an all-time high. Heart disease, high cholesterol and other medical issues are also reaching epidemic proportions primarily because of the food that people are eating.

High carb, high sugar, and high fat foods will destroy your body over time and make you gain weight. Your body can't process refined sugar. It doesn't break down refined sugar and use it for fuel, so that sugar is converted into fat.

Natural sugars are broken down by the body and converted into fuel. So just cutting out refined sugar and eating foods that contain natural sugar, like fruit, can make a huge difference in your health and have a big impact on your weight.

What you eat is more important that how much you eat. When you are eating healthy food that provides fuel for your body you don't need to deprive yourself of food in order to lose weight.

Starving yourself won't make you lose weight. Only changing the foods that you're eating can do that.

It can be difficult to change how you eat. Most people have a long list of excuses to rationalize why they can't eat healthy.

Some of the most common excuses people give for eating a terrible diet are:

- Healthy food isn't tasty.

- I can't cook.

- I'm too busy to cook for every meal and fast food is just easier.

- I'm on a budget.

- There's no point in cooking for just 1 or 2 people.

Do any of those excuses sound familiar? But that's all they are – excuses. There is no reason you can't eat healthy food and change your life.

These powerful eating habits will teach you how to build a new and healthy relationship with food that won't require you to be a gourmet chef, have unlimited funds to spend on food, or never have a tasty treat.

Eating Habit #1 – Cut Down on The Carbs

One of the easiest and most effective ways to lose belly fat is to cut carbs and change the carbs that you do eat.

Modern diets use a lot of carbs as fillers. Pasta, bread, rice and other carb heavy foods are staples that people at every meal. But those carbs are causing you to gain weight and can make it impossible to lose fat.

How carbs make you fat

When you eat carbs, they are broken down by the body into glucose. When your blood has too much glucose in it, the body turns that glucose into fat and stores it for extra energy.

But that fat builds up, and builds up more when you keep eating carbs and your body doesn't need the extra energy.

That's what makes you gain weight.

Pasta, bread and other foods made from refined flour are almost entirely made of starch, which is quickly converted to glucose and then is turned into fat.

Small amounts of fat are deposited into your liver for storage but the rest has nowhere to go so the body deposits it wherever there is room like your arms, your belly, your thighs and so on.

Healthy carbs vs. unhealthy carbs

Not all carbs are unhealthy.

Your body does need carbs to function effectively. Your brain also needs carbs in order to keep working. But you should be eating healthy carbs instead of unhealthy ones and eating only small amounts of them.

Healthy carbs come from natural sources like vegetables and some fruits. Fruits also contain natural sugar so they should be eaten in small amounts.

Eating healthy carbs will give you the energy that you need without causing weight gain. A combination of protein and healthy carbs will turn your body into a fat burning machine because your body will burn all that stored fat for energy.

Getting into the habit of eating healthy carbs instead of carbs from bread, rice or pasta will keep you healthy and help you lose fat.

Cutting carbs out of your diet can be tough, especially if you are on a tight budget. High carb foods are usually much cheaper than healthy fresh fruits and vegetables.

Here are some easy ways that you can start cutting carbs out of your diet without dramatically changing how you eat:

- Use lettuce instead of bread for a sandwich or burger. All you really need is a wrapper for your burger or sandwich so use lettuce instead of high carb bread.

- Eat more eggs. Eggs are a cheap source of protein that anyone can afford. Hard-boil some for quick and easy snacks.

- Swap pasta noodles for zoodles. You can make noodles from vegetables like zucchini so that you can still enjoy your favorite pasta dishes without high carb pasta.

Eating Habit #2 – Stop Drinking Soda

Soda is one of the worst things that you can put in your body. If you want to lose fat and be healthy you need to stop drinking it.

Regular soda is high in calories and has a massive amount of sugar.

Diet sodas are even worse, and studies have proven that the artificial sweeteners in diet soda can lead to weight gain. It can be hard to give up soda but you will feel better and lose weight if you stop drinking it.

Why soda is the worst drink

There are lots of unhealthy drinks out there but soda is the worst because of the way that the high amounts of sugar and artificial sweeteners affect the body.

Eating or drinking a lot of sugar will wreak havoc on your body. Your body has to work even harder to break down the sugar and it will get stored in the body as fat.

The body uses insulin to break down sugar, so the more sugar you eat or drink the more insulin your body will produce. That causes too much insulin in the body. When the body has too much insulin it will make your blood sugar drop and can lead to poor concentration, fatigue, and other problems.

Diet soda is even worse. The artificial sweeteners used in diet soda have been linked to metabolic disorder and even to diabetes.

Healthy alternatives to soda

The best thing to drink is water. But if you just can't force yourself to drink plain water there are lots of ways that you can make water more appealing.

If you like the carbonation in sodas try drinking sparkling water.

You can add some cucumber slices or lemon juice to the sparkling water for a tasty and refreshing drink. Or you can mix a small amount of natural fruit juice with some sparkling water to create a fruit spritzer.

Herbal tea is another great alternative to soda because you can drink it hot or cold.

Most people drink soda because it's easy to find everywhere and it's usually pretty cheap.

Here are some easy ways to avoid falling into the trap of drinking soda just because it's what is available:

- Get a water bottle. Having a water bottle with you will ensure that you have a healthy drink with you no matter where you go.

- Bring a tea bag to restaurants. Most restaurants won't charge you for hot water so instead of ordering a soda, just ask for some hot water and have tea.

- Stash some water at the office and in your car. If you have water within reach you won't be tempted to get a soda from a vending machine or at the store.

Read This FIRST - Your FREE BONUS

FOR A LIMITED TIME ONLY – You can get Linda's best-selling book *"Quick & Easy Weight Loss: 97 Scientifically Proven Tips Even For Those With Busy Schedules!"* absolutely FREE!

People who have read this bonus book as well, have seen the best weight loss results, and have quickly & easily improved overall fitness levels – so it is *highly recommended* that you get this bonus book.

Don't forget that it is free right now, but won't be for very long!

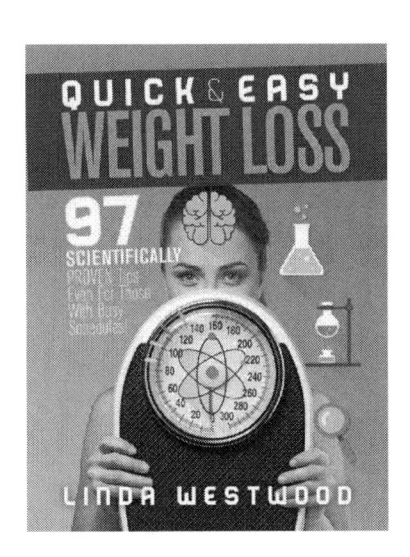

Get your free copy at:

TopFitnessAdvice.com/Bonus

Eating Habit #3 – Eat Vegetables with Every Meal

Remember when you were young and your parents told you to eat all your vegetables?

That's still good advice.

You should be eating probably double the amount of vegetables that you are eating every day. In fact, most of the carbs that you eat during the day should be coming from vegetables. You should be having at least one serving of vegetables with every meal, even breakfast.

Why vegetables are so important

Vegetables contain the vitamins and minerals that your body needs to stay healthy and work efficiently.

They are low in calories and carbs and yet they are filling. Because they are low in calories you can eat a lot of them and still not gain weight.

The carbs in vegetables are easier for your body to break down and use than the carbs in things like pasta or bread. That means that your body will quickly break down the carbs in the vegetables that you eat and use those carbs for fuel instead of storing them as fat.

The vitamins and minerals in vegetables will help your body repair damaged tissue, keep muscles strong, and keep your body working the way it's supposed to. Vegetables keep your body in balance.

Try new vegetables

One of the biggest reasons why people say they don't eat vegetables is that they find vegetables boring. But there are hundreds of vegetables that you're not eating. Most people only try the same 9-10 vegetables they have been eating since they were children.

In order to make vegetables more appealing try some different types of vegetables.

Eating seasonally is a fabulous way to try different kinds of vegetables as well as save money because seasonal vegetables are always cheaper than vegetables that have to be shipped in from other places.

Visit a local farmer's market and check out the many different kinds of seasonal vegetables available. You can also join a farm share program where you pay a fee and the farm delivers farm fresh seasonal vegetables to your door.

Here are a few easy ways to get more vegetables into your daily diet:

- Swap vegetables for pasta and rice with dinner.

- Eat a different kind of salad every day for lunch.

- Serve vegetables and healthy dip as an appetizer.

- Keep a container of cut up vegetables at work for a quick snack.

- Throw some spinach into your morning omelet.

- Make a vegetable soup.

Eating Habit #4 – Drink More Water

How much water do you drink each day?

Chances are it's not enough. Studies have shown that people underestimate how much water they should be drinking each day.

The body is 70% water and unless you are replenishing the fluids the body loses each day you won't be healthy. Drinking water also is essential if you want to lose weight.

Water and weight loss

Water is critically important when it comes to weight loss and fat loss.

Drinking water will help flush out all the toxins from your cells which will keep your body healthy. Drinking water will also make you feel full which will lead to eating less and eventually weight loss.

Drinking a glass of water before each meal will make you feel full faster so that you don't want to eat as much. Drinking water instead of having an afternoon snack will make you feel full without eating a high calorie snack.

Drinking water will also help your muscles stay strong, and the more muscle you have the more calories you will burn.

Water and the brain

Drinking water is essential for healthy brain function. When you are dehydrated you will find it hard to focus and you may be sleepy.

When that happens, your brain will tell your body to have a snack in order to wake up and get through the day. That's when you will reach for sugary carb-laden snacks and drinks that will give you a boost of energy. But water is the best booster in the world.

Instead of reaching for a candy bar when you're tired or can't focus on work, reach for a bottle of water instead.

Water infused with vegetables or fruit will give you a quick jump start so that you will have the energy to get through your day, go workout, and take care of all your responsibilities.

The biggest reason why people don't drink enough water is that they think it's not convenient. But it's easy to keep water with you all day, if you just get creative and invest in a few simple tools. Use these tips to drink more water every day:

- Keep a pitcher of water in the fridge so it's ice cold and ready to go all the time.

- Put some cucumber slices, lemon wedges, or berries into an infusion pitcher to make tasty flavored water.

- Buy a water bottle and carry it with you wherever you go.

- Drink a glass of water or tea before every meal.

Eating Habit #5 - Cut Down on Caffeine

One of the things causing you to have excess belly fat could be your daily caffeine consumption. High calorie coffee drinks contain a lot more calories than most people think.

A large coffee drink can have 1000 calories or more. But it's not just high calorie fancy coffee drinks that can cause belly fat.

Most people think that caffeine will help them lose weight because it is a stimulant but that's not the case. Coffee or foods that are high in caffeine can actually cause you to gain belly fat. And that belly fat can be extremely hard to get rid of because it's caused by a hormone, called Cortisol.

Cortisol and belly fat

Cortisol is a hormone that your body pumps out when you are under a lot of stress. Not getting enough sleep can trigger Cortisol production in the body. So can stress at work or dealing with a lot of stress at home. But caffeine also causes the body to produce Cortisol because it stimulates the brain and nervous system.

If you drink too much caffeine your body has a "fight or flight" response the same way it would if you were in a life or death situation.

The body starts pumping out adrenaline and Cortisol.

When there's too much Cortisol in your body, the body will hang onto fat and store it, usually around your belly, in case you need to burn it for energy later. But when you don't use it for energy it just stays around your midsection. And every time you have too much caffeine your belly gets bigger and bigger thanks to Cortisol.

Cutting caffeine

That doesn't mean that you need to give up your daily morning coffee though. Just cutting down on the amount of caffeine that you consume each day is enough to lower the Cortisol levels in your body.

If you need your morning cup of coffee have just one cup, then switch to a lower caffeine drink like decaf coffee or tea.

Don't drink caffeine after noon. Don't drink sodas either because many sodas have more caffeine than a cup of coffee. There are other ways that you can lower your Cortisol levels too, which help you lose belly fat.

These activities can help lower your Cortisol levels:

- Yoga
- Meditation
- Walking
- Gentle Exercise
- Napping

Eating Habit #6 - Snack Smart

You'd be surprised how many calories you can rack up each day snacking.

Snacking is one of the most common reasons why people gain weight, especially around the midsection.

If you work at a job where you are sitting all day and you spend a lot of the day snacking those extra calories can add up to excess belly fat in a very short amount of time.

Eating frequently throughout the day can be good for weight loss, but only if you eat the right things.

Six small meals a day

One of the best ways to lose weight is to eat six small meals each day instead of three large meals.

Ideally you should eat a snack size meal every few hours. But that doesn't mean you should be popping open a bag of chips every couple hours or eating candy bars.

What you should be eating are protein heavy snacks like cheese or eggs with some vegetables and maybe some fruit.

Healthy snacking can be a major fat buster because it turns your body into fat burning machine.

Protein power

When you eat primarily protein you will burn fat faster for several reasons.

One of those reasons is that protein rebuilds muscle, and the more muscle you have the more calories you burn. Even when you are just sitting you will burn more calories if you have more muscle.

Protein also makes you feel full so that you don't eat as much. A small protein rich snack will keep you full for hours, but a carb heavy snack will make you feel hungry again quickly and all those carbs will end up stored in your body as fat.

The secret to eating healthy protein snacks instead of carb heavy snacks is preparation. You may not be able to go cook a burger when you want a snack but you can bring a couple of hardboiled eggs with you to work, to the gym, or anywhere else you go.

Protein bars are convenient and can stay in a desk drawer or a purse indefinitely.

Here are some other easy ways to keep protein snacks handy:

- Beef jerky is pure protein and easy to store.

- Make a salad in a jar and store it in the office refrigerator for a quick and healthy snack.

- Cook some eggs, cheese and spinach in a muffin tin so that you have small snack size frittatas and keep them in the freezer. Microwave a couple for a quick protein snack.

Eating Habit #7 – Swap Foods

Food swaps are a great way to change the way that you eat without sacrificing the foods that you love.

If you avoid dieting because you don't want to have to deprive yourself of things you really like to eat you can use simple swaps to make those foods healthier.

When you swap out some of the worst ingredients in the dishes you love you can cut calories, carbs, and unhealthy sugar, which will help you burn that belly fat and feel better.

Why food swapping works so well

Food swaps are one of the easiest ways to change your diet because in most dishes you can't even tell that one food was swapped for another.

In some dishes the food that is swapped is even more delicious than the original ingredient in the dish. Food swaps also mean that you and your family can all eat the same dishes you already enjoy. You don't have to make two separate meals at every meal just so that you can lose weight. Everyone can eat the same dish and enjoy the same healthy food.

Food swaps make it easier to eat healthy. Your family may not even realize that some of their favorite dishes contain food swaps.

Use these easy food swaps in your favorite dishes to dial up the protein, dial down the carbs, and burn belly fat:

- Swap Greek yogurt for sour cream: Greek yogurt is low in calories and packed with healthy protein.

- Swap Zoodles for Pasta Noodles: Zoodles, or noodles made from zucchini, are very trendy right now. They're also super healthy. Zoodles are low in calories and contain natural healthy carbs instead of carbs from starchy refined flour that you will find in pasta noodles. You can cut zoodles yourself or buy an inexpensive noodle maker that will make them for you.

- Swap cheese for bread: Instead of using bread to make a deli meat sandwich, use sliced cheese. Put a little mayonnaise on a slice of cheese, layer on some deli meat and top it with a slice of cheese for a snack of pure protein that will zap belly fat and keep you full.

- Swap nuts for chips: When you just have to have to a crunchy snack, eat some healthy nuts like peanuts or cashews instead of chips. Nuts can be high in calories like chips but at least they are packed with protein instead of empty calories. Cashews are also very good for your teeth.

- Eat vegetables instead of candy: Splurge and buy a tray full of fresh cut veggies to eat with a Greek yogurt dip. You'd spend just as much on candy or ice cream and the vegetables are much healthier.

Spend money on healthy foods and snacks instead of on junk food.

Eating Habit #8 - Skip Dessert

This habit can be tough, especially if you love dessert. But getting in the habit of skipping dessert can help you lose fat and maintain a healthy weight.

Dessert doesn't have to be something you eat every day. In fact, dessert is better when it's something you don't have all the time.

Desserts are often high in fat, sugar, calories and carbs so eating dessert all the time really packs on the pounds.

Often people think it's fine to treat themselves to dessert, but why treat yourself with food?

Food is fuel for your body. Look for other things to reward yourself with.

Dessert is a once in a while food

That doesn't mean you have to skip your favorite holiday dessert or not have birthday cake on your birthday. But it does mean that on a day-to-day basis you should just skip it.

Don't keep sweets in the house and don't prepare dessert as a part of dinner.

If you want a snack a few hours after dinner, have some vegetables with hummus or some nuts or even a piece of fruit.

The natural sugar in fruit is much easier for your body to break down than refined sugar.

You don't have to go hungry. You just have to make different food choices. Before long you won't even miss dessert.

Treats don't have to be food

Instead of treating yourself to dessert every day put aside the money that you would spend on dessert and once a week buy yourself a book, or take a class, or go see a movie.

Try a yoga class or buy some hobby materials. Stop rewarding yourself with food. You will get a lot more value out of doing something for yourself that doesn't involve food.

Buy a new journal or a new CD. Invest in yourself by learning a new skill or having some fun that isn't associated with food. You will feel better, have more fun, and you never know what new sport or hobby you might find that you enjoy.

Start by cutting out dessert just two nights each week and slowly work up to giving up dessert altogether.

Here are some fun things you can try with the money you save on dessert:

- Buy a new bike and go on a bike ride with your kids.

- Buy a pair of cozy slippers.

- Buy a water bottle so that you will start drinking more water.

- Visit a local farmer's market and buy some fresh local produce.

- Buy some gardening books and learn to grow your own vegetables.

- Take your partner to the movies.

Eating Habit #9 - Cut Out Refined Sugar

Refined sugar is something that has been proven to cause belly fat. That's because refined sugar is a simple carbohydrate.

Complex carbohydrates are the carbs that give you energy. Simple carbs are just empty calories that end up as fat in the body because they have no nutritional value.

Most people don't even realize how much refined sugar they are eating every day because they don't realize that nearly every prepared food or restaurant food contains at least some refined sugar and some foods contain huge amounts of it.

Hidden in plain sight

If you think that just because you don't put refined sugar in your coffee or eat sugary snacks you're safe from refined sugar you're wrong.

Every day foods that you wouldn't think contain sugar actually do have sugar in them. Things like spaghetti sauce, salad dressing, canned vegetables, yogurt, crackers, breads and other foods.

Over the years, food manufacturers started adding more and more sugar to their products so that people would buy them.

Prepared foods like boxed mashed potatoes, stuffing and other foods also have hidden sugar in them. Most people are eating 3x the amount of sugar they should be eating daily without even realizing it.

How to cut your sugar consumption

First you need to stop drinking soda, fruit juice with added sugar, and fancy coffee drinks that are packed with sugar.

Smoothies also contain added sugar, even though they are supposed to be healthy.

The next thing you need to do is start-preparing food from scratch. It may seem daunting but it's really not as hard as you think.

Preparing your own food from raw ingredients will ensure that you are not eating a lot of sugar that you don't want to be eating. Also start reading food labels closely to find out if they have hidden sugar.

If you aren't feeling secure enough to start cooking from scratch then look for diabetic friendly foods when you shop.

Diabetic foods will have lower sugar content and no added sugar.

Other ways you can cut your intake of refined sugar include:

- Switch to a natural sugar substitute. Use that for coffee, baking, or cereal.

- Use natural, locally grown honey as a sweetener. Honey has a wide range of health benefits.

- Drink water instead of bottled tea and soda.

- Look for dark chocolate bars, which have lower sugar content.

- Eat more fruit and naturally sweet foods.

- Make your own sauces and dips.

- Buy unsweetened plain yogurt and flavor it yourself with berries and spices.

Eating Habit #10 - Eat More Fat

That sounds crazy right?

For years people have been told that low fat diets are the only healthy diets and that eating fat makes you fat. But that's not the case.

In fact, not eating any fat just makes you hungry and it actually makes it harder for your body to burn fat. The body needs fat in order to function.

However, that doesn't mean you can go out and start eating cupcakes all day long. You need to eat healthy fats in order to lose fat.

When you eat healthy fats you will feel full longer and you won't eat as much. Your body will also function better and burn more fat for energy, which will help you lose fat.

Healthy fat vs. unhealthy fat

There really are healthy fats that you should be eating, even though that might sound too good to be true.

The fats in foods like yogurt, avocadoes, nuts, seeds and oils like olive oil are healthy and you should be eating more of them. About ten percent of your daily calories should come from healthy fats if you want to lose weight.

Diets like the Mediterranean diet, which are high in protein and healthy fats, are strongly recommended by doctors because they provide the protein and fat that many people are lacking in their daily diets. Even the fat in some meat like bacon can be healthy if you don't overdo it.

Low fat is making you fat

Low fat diet food is something that you should avoid.

Foods that are advertised as low fat really just use chemical sweeteners and other additives to make the food taste good while removing things like cream and butter, which are healthy fats.

Those chemical additives contribute directly to weight gain and belly fat. It's much better to eat foods with natural fat in them than to eat supposed low fat food if you want to burn belly fat.

So stop denying yourself healthy food that contains fat. Those foods usually contain high amounts of protein as well as healthy fat.

Here are some of the natural healthy fats you should be eating more of:

- Fish
- Nuts
- Olive Oil
- Butter
- Eggs
- Avocados
- Nut Butters like Peanut Butter or Almond Butter

Eating Habit #11- Eat More Protein

You've probably seen the many different high protein diets in the news like Atkins, Paleo and so on.

The one thing that these diets all have in common is that they encourage people to eat more protein to lose weight. And you know what? That's because eating protein does lead to fat loss.

Protein burns fat it's true

Study after study has shown that increasing the amount of protein that you eat will boost your metabolism and push your body to burn stored fat as fuel.

You don't need to follow a fad diet to lose fat. Just double the amount of protein that you are eating and cut down on carbs. You will start losing inches almost immediately.

When you eat more protein, you will actually eat less of everything else. Protein is what makes you feel full. Eating protein will make it easy to lose weight without feeling deprived or hungry.

Not all carbs are equal

You will still need to eat some carbs. Humans need carbs in their diets. But the carbs that you eat should come from vegetables and not from refined flour-based foods like bread and pasta.

Double the protein that you're eating, and cut out bread and pasta. Just those simple dietary changes will help you burn fat and lose weight.

One of the most common excuses that people give for not eating more protein is that protein rich meats and other foods can be expensive and not practical for someone on a budget.

The sad truth is that pasta and bread are cheap food that even people on a tight budget can afford.

You can't afford to eat bad food

But what is the price of staying overweight?

How do you put a price on your health?

The bottom line is that you can't afford not to eat more protein.

Most people get about 10% of their daily calories from protein but that number should be more like 35%. The amount of calories that you eat isn't as important as the amount of protein that you're eating.

That's why people who follow the Paleo diet eat high calorie meats with every meal and still lose weight.

Some easy ways to sneak more protein into diet and cut down on carbs are:

- Eat more eggs. Eggs are inexpensive and pure protein. You can cook them dozens of different ways so that you don't get sick of them.

- Stock up on protein bars. Not all protein has to come from meat or cheese. Many stores routinely put protein bars on sale. Stock up on your favorite protein bars when they are on sale so you will have plenty of protein rich snacks. Just make sure the bars are low in carbs and sugar.

- Cook ahead. A major stumbling block for people trying to eat more protein is having to cook meat or protein at every meal. But you can use a slow cooker to prepare food in advance. Or mix up eggs, bacon, spinach and cheese in a bowl and pour the mixture into a muffin tin and bake. Freeze the egg "muffins" and you can microwave one whenever you need a quick meal or snack.

Eating Habit #12 – Eat Breakfast

Did you eat breakfast this morning?

If not, you should be starting tomorrow.

Your parents probably told you that breakfast is the most important meal of the day. And they were right! Studies have proven that there are very real benefits to eating breakfast every day.

Not eating can make you fat

When you eat breakfast you are kick starting your metabolism to burn more calories. Your body needs fuel in the morning. If you don't give it fuel it goes into starvation mode.

When your body thinks it is starving it will hang onto every calorie and every bit of fat in case you go hungry for a long time. So not eating actually makes you gain weight.

What you eat is important too. You should eat a protein rich breakfast to give you the energy that you need to face the day and to keep you full until lunch. Eating in the morning triggers the production of Leptin in the body.

Leptin is what makes you feel full. When your body has enough Leptin and your stomach feels full you won't be tempted to hit the bagel shop or vending machine for a carb heavy snack in the middle of the morning.

I'm too busy for breakfast

This is the number one excuse that people use to justify skipping breakfast. But it's also a lie. Breakfast doesn't have to take a long time to cook or be food that you have to sit down and eat.

When you have the time to cook eggs and bacon is a great breakfast. But if you are pressed for time yogurt or some cheese is a good breakfast too.

Protein bars are the ultimate portable healthy breakfast for people who barely have time to make it to work.

Here are some quick and easy breakfast ideas that even the busiest person can make time for:

- Greek yogurt is high in protein and easy to grab on your way out the door. Keep a spoon in your bag or in the car.

- Hard-boiled eggs are easy to take on the go and pack a powerful protein punch. They are also great for snacks.

- Fruit and fruit smoothies are not the best choice but they are better than a bagel or a sugary coffee drink. The natural sugars in fruit are better for you than refined sugar and fruit is full of vitamins and minerals.

- Go veggie. Salads aren't just for lunch. At night prepare a salad with healthy veggies, hard-boiled eggs, and some bacon. Grab the salad on your way out the door and eat breakfast at your desk.

Eating Habit #13 – Use a Crockpot

Using a crockpot or a slow cooker is a fantastic way to eat healthier. Crockpots are very inexpensive and they last for a long time. Best of all they make it easy to eat healthy.

What is a crockpot?

A crockpot is a small kitchen appliance that uses low heat to slow cook food in a ceramic basin. It has a timer so that you can set it to cook for a number of hours. It can be left on to cook while you are at work or while you are asleep. Investing in a crockpot is one of the best things you can do to eat healthy.

A crockpot saves time and money

Using a crockpot makes it easier to avoid unhealthy food like fast food or pre-packaged food because the food is ready when you're ready for it.

It's the ultimate healthy fast food. Instead of running through the drive through for dinner you can come home to a perfectly cooked healthy meal. Or you can start off the day with a healthy hot breakfast if you put the ingredients in the crockpot when you go to bed and turn it on. A crockpot also saves money.

If you want to eat more protein but can't afford pricey cuts of meat you can buy cheaper cuts of meat and cook them in a crockpot.

Usually the cheaper cuts of meat are kind of tough and not very good. But slow cooked in a crockpot with vegetables and broth they turn into succulent pieces of meat that are delicious and cheap.

Anyone can cook with a crockpot

Even if you aren't the greatest cook in the world you can make delicious meals in a crockpot. All you have to do is put the ingredients in the pot and let them cook.

Almost anything can be cooked in a crockpot from soups and stews to rice or dessert. You can even use it to make delicious drinks and punches.

Check out some of these easy to make but healthy crockpot dishes:

- Oatmeal with Apples and Cinnamon
- Shredded Beef or Chicken with Vegetables
- Lasagna
- Braised Lamb
- Lamb or Beef Stew
- Queso Dip
- Pumpkin Pudding
- Short Ribs
- Sweet Potato Mash
- Turkey Chili
- Roast Chicken

Eating Habit #14 – Grow Your Own Vegetables

Growing your own vegetables is an easy way to get the healthy food you should be eating without spending a fortune.

Most people don't grow their own food because they think that it's expensive or difficult to grow vegetables.

But it's much cheaper than buying vegetables at local markets and you can get better quality vegetables from your own backyard!

I don't have space to grow anything

It's a myth that you need a huge yard or a lot of land in order to grow vegetables.

You can grow vegetables in planters on a patio, or in pots inside the house, or in window gardens. Some creative city dwellers have even grown vegetables in old 2 liter bottles cut in half and attached to the outside wall of their apartments. Container gardening is easy and cheap.

I don't know what vegetables to grow

It's easy to find out what types of vegetables grow well in your area.

Your local gardening store or home improvement store will be able to answer your questions when you are choosing what to grow.

They can also help you get set up to start growing your own vegetables.

Imagine eating fresh vegetables from your yard with your dinner every night!

Community gardens with neighbors

If you don't want to put in all the work of growing vegetables yourself and you have a little room you can get together with your neighbors and create a community garden.

When you share a community garden everyone helps out with the work in order to get a share of the vegetables. Lots of people would jump at the chance to grow their own fresh vegetables. Ask your neighbors to see if they want to start a community garden with you.

Here are some easy ways to start growing your own vegetables so that you can eat healthier and save money:

- Start with one or two vegetables that you like. Pick lettuce and tomatoes, or cucumbers and squash, or whatever vegetables you like the best. Starting small will give you a chance to get used to gardening without overwhelming you.

- Use simple containers. You can use wood pallets, the plastic troughs that catch rain in rain gutters, or basic planting boxes to start growing vegetables. You can even build a small square garden with a few pieces of lumber.

- Track your progress. Keep track of how well your garden is growing by taking photos and videos of the plants as they grow. That way you can see what you're doing right and what you're doing wrong.

Eating Habit #15 – Drink Green Tea

One of the best things you can do to lose fat is drink green tea. Really, that's all you need to do. Enjoy a cup of delicious green tea and you will lose fat.

That's because green tea is packed with antioxidants and other natural elements that will boost your metabolism. Enjoy some green tea instead of coffee throughout the day and your metabolism will keep burning fat all day long.

How green tea causes weight loss

Green tea is one of the healthiest things that you can eat or drink. It has a powerful combination of antioxidants and low amounts of caffeine. There's not enough caffeine to make you jittery. There's just enough to give your metabolism a little boost.

The antioxidants help repair damaged cells in the body and keep your body working efficiently. When your body is working efficiently it will burn fat for energy and you will lose fat.

Drinking tea means drinking more water

Another benefit that comes with drinking green tea is that you're drinking more water.

Water is essential for weight loss. When you drink green tea all the toxins are washed out of your cells which helps your body function better and helps flush out your body.

The more tea and water you drink the more fat you will lose.

Make green tea part of your day

Green tea can be enjoyed hot or cold, and you can add berries and other things to it if you want to add more flavors.

There are endless ways to get more green tea into your daily diet.

You can make iced green tea and leave it at the office so that you have a healthy drink waiting for you each day. Or you can take a break from your work to make some delicious hot green tea.

Here are some creative ways to drink more green tea:

- Use it in smoothies. If you make smoothies for breakfast replace the water in the smoothie with green tea.

- Get a tea tumbler. You can buy travel cups that have a slot for tea so that you can easily make tea all day long just by adding water.

- Cook with it. Did you know that you can use green tea to flavor desserts and breads? Just replace the water in the recipe with green tea. You can even use green tea in homemade salad dressings.

- Carry some green tea with you. Put a few green tea bags in your wallet or bag. When you go out to eat ask for some hot water instead of coffee or soda and have some green tea instead.

Eating Habit #16 – Drink Apple Cider Vinegar Every Day

What? Drink vinegar? It's true.

Apple cider vinegar has been used for centuries as a bit of a cure-all because it has a lot of different healing properties.

One of the things that it can do is regulate blood sugar and burn fat. It tastes a little gross at first but the benefits make the taste worth it.

Apple cider vinegar gave roman soldiers strength

Most people don't know this but the drink that Roman soldiers drank every day and took with them on their famous marches was made from Apple Cider Vinegar. It was called Posca.

Apple Cider Vinegar was mixed with honey and some plain water and Roman soldiers drank it to stay strong and lean.

Apple Cider Vinegar also is a great energy boost when you need some extra energy for a workout.

Apple cider vinegar and weight loss

So how does apple cider vinegar help with weight loss?

It does a lot of amazing things for the body. One thing it does is help your body break down protein and use it effectively.

So when you start eating more protein to lose fat and you drink apple cider vinegar you are turning your body into a fat burning machine.

Apple cider vinegar also regulates blood sugar. This means that you won't crave carbs and sugar so much. You also won't experience any energy crashes that leave you wanting snacks to give you energy.

How to drink apple cider vinegar

You can't drink straight apple cider vinegar.

Well you can, but it tastes terrible and it's very harsh by itself.

The best way to drink apple cider vinegar is to put a teaspoon or two into a bottle of water and shake it. Then drink the water. The water dilutes the taste.

You can also add a little honey like the Romans did. Some of the other benefits of drinking apple cider vinegar everyday are:

- Apple cider vinegar can lower your risk of cardiovascular disease.

- Apple cider vinegar is an antimicrobial and antibacterial agent that can kill germs and bacteria in your body.

- Apple cider vinegar can even lower your risk of some types of cancer.

- Apple cider vinegar can get rid of heartburn.

- Apple cider vinegar can get rid of muscle cramps.

Eating Habit #17 – Plan Your Meals

How many times each week do you get fast food or pizza because you just don't want to think about what to have for dinner again?

How many times this week alone have you gone out for lunch because you didn't plan ahead and have a healthy lunch ready to bring to work? Too many, if you're like most people.

Planning meals is an easy habit to get into that can help you lose a lot of weight. Most people don't plan a menu for the week because they think that it's too much work. But when you plan your meals you can create meals that will maximize fat burning and give your body the fuel it needs.

Protein rich meals that include healthy carbs don't just happen. You need to plan them.

When you plan ahead you can buy the ingredients you need and even prepare meals ahead of time. That will keep you from grabbing fast food on the way from work because you're tired or because you can't decide what to make for dinner.

Creating healthy meals

When you are planning meals you should aim to have 60% of the meal consist of protein. 30% of the meal should be vegetables or healthy carbs. 10% of the meal should be healthy fats. Using these figures as a guideline you can plan out healthy meals that will help you lose weight and burn fat.

If you are crunched for time you can plan for that and prepare meals and snacks that are healthy ahead of time. A little time spent planning can lead to dramatic weight loss that will help you meet your goals and stay at a healthy weight.

Planning balanced and healthy meals will also teach your kids healthy eating habits that they will use for the rest of their lives. Studies have shown that kids will repeat the eating habits they learn as children.

Trying new things

When you plan meals, you can also get more creative with what you eat.

Instead of pulling out some frozen chicken again because you have to cook something you might find that you really like trying new and exciting dishes that will make meals more interesting.

Here are some tips that will help you get started planning meals and snacks:

- Make an appointment to plan meals. Set aside an hour or two on a weekend or before you shop for groceries to plan out meals. Write it on your schedule and set a reminder on your phone or tablet.

- Print off a weekly calendar. Write on the calendar what meals and snacks you're going to have. Then post it on the fridge or in a central place so you and your family will know what meals you're having each day.

- Coordinate your shopping list and meal plan. As you plan the meal on a sheet of paper jot down all the ingredients you need for that meal. Use that jotted list as the basis for your shopping list. That way you can be sure you have everything you need.

- Be flexible. Some days you might have to swap one meal for another one based on time constraints, weather, or other factors. It only takes a few minutes to change the menu around. When unexpected things happen don't order out. Just swap meals that you have already planned.

Eating Habit #18 – Make Your Own Lunches

Taking your own lunch to work or school will save you money. It also will keep you eating healthy and not indulging in fast food or restaurant lunches. Taking your own lunch is a fantastic way to lose weight.

Lunchtime blues

When you're working in an office all day it can be very tempting to get fast food lunches or go out with coworkers for lunch. But four or five days a week of high calorie and high fat food can make you put on weight very quickly.

Going out with friends for lunch once in a while is fine, as long as you choose relatively healthy food, but bringing your own lunch is something you should do most of the time.

Creating tasty lunches

If you don't choose fun and creative lunches, chances are good that they will sit in the refrigerator until you throw them away. When you're at work lunch is a big deal. If the food isn't tasty or if it's boring you won't want to eat it.

Luckily there are a lot of fun options for low carb healthy lunches that you can take to work. Some of them need to be refrigerated but others don't.

Invest in a small cooler that you can use to keep your lunch in so that you have more options when it comes to what foods you can bring to work.

Choose healthy carbs

You will probably need some healthy carbs to keep you going through a long workday. That's fine as long as you choose healthy carbs.

Most of the meal should be protein, but you can add some healthy carbs from vegetables and even some fruit if you crave something sweet.

Salty, crunchy nuts are a good addition to brown bag lunches because they will satisfy your cravings and give you a nice protein boost.

If you have no idea what to make for brown bag lunches that don't include peanut butter sandwiches here are some easy to make but delicious low carb lunches you can start taking to work:

- Pepperoni and cheese. You can get the best part of a pizza without the crust. Bring some sliced mozzarella cheese and pepperoni for lunch and heat them up together so that the cheese is just a little melted. Or put them on some vegetables.

- Salads. There are dozens of different types of salads you can bring for lunch. Add hard-boiled eggs, chicken, ham, or other proteins to the salad to add some substance if a simple salad will leave you hungry. You can find some ingenious ways to carry salad fixings to work online so that the salad ingredients stay fresh.

- Soups. Hearty soups are a great choice for lunch. Just check the carb count and be sure there's no added sugar in the soup.

- Cheese. A couple ounces of sliced cheese is delicious and satisfying. You can also bring some cheese as a snack.

- Burgers. A classic lunch of a couple of burgers without buns and a salad is a good choice too. Cook the burgers ahead of time and heat them in the microwave. You can shake things up by trying lamb, buffalo, or turkey burgers instead of beef.

Eating Habit #19 - Make Your Own Convenience Food

Pre-packaged food is unhealthy, but it's definitely convenient.

That's why it's so much easier to pick up pre-packaged food than it is to make your own healthy food. But relying on pre-packaged food is part of the reason why you gained weight. And it's going to prevent you from losing fat.

Luckily there is a convenient alternative. Make your own convenience food.

Healthy food can be convenient too

They key to making healthy convenience food is to plan ahead. You can make food that is healthy and package it so that it's easy to cook or easy to grab when you're in a hurry.

When you're hungry and pressed for time even if you have the best intentions to eat healthy you're going to be tempted by the fast food drive thru or a quick food like pizza.

But you can create healthy options for those times when you need a quick dinner or a quick snack or a quick breakfast so that you won't be reaching for the take-out menu.

Healthy choices can be delicious

After you have been eating healthy food for a bit you will notice that the snack foods and fast food that you used to like doesn't taste good to you anymore.

Once you stop eating high carb foods, fried foods, and sugary foods your body won't want those foods anymore. Instead your body will crave the healthy low carb foods you have been eating.

How to make healthy food convenient

Expanding your food horizons and being prepared makes it easier to make healthy food convenient.

Invest in a crockpot and some good take along containers that can be used often. When you have the right equipment, it will be easy to make food to bring with you instead of buying food on the go.

A portable water bottle and a travel mug are also essential. With a portable tea mug, you can make tea and coffee to drink instead of buying sugary high-priced coffee drinks.

Buy a water bottle with a filter so even tap water will taste like spring water.

Here are some other ways to make healthy food and snacks that are convenient:

- Cook on the weekends. If you know you are tired and don't want to cook when you get home from work pick one day on the weekend to cook for the week. Cook several meals. Put them in containers and freeze them. You can heat one up for dinner during the week.

- Portion out your food ahead of time. Take things like burgers, chicken breasts, sauces, vegetables and pasta and put them in individual portion containers. Keep them in the fridge or the freezer. You can grab them to put into a lunch sack to take to work or heat up a quick dinner when you're pressed for time.

- Create your own healthy snacks. Choose healthy foods like pretzels, nuts, seeds, and dried fruit to make your own snack mix. Portion the mix into individual bags and put a bag in your car, in your purse, in your desk at work or anywhere that you usually get hungry.

- Buy healthy packaged food. There are some healthy options when it comes to convenience food. Individual cheese wedges, yogurt, and fruit are all healthy snacks that you can buy. Pre-cut vegetable trays and fruit assortments are worth the money because they give you healthy and fast snack options.

Eating Habit #20 – Eat More

Eat more to lose weight? That sounds crazy but it's true.

Most people eat food that is full of empty calories and that's why they gain weight. If you want to lose fat and build muscle you need to eat more.

The catch is that you have to be eating the right kinds of foods if you want to lose fat.

Starvation mode

Restricting calories isn't enough to cause fat loss. If it was, losing weight wouldn't be so hard.

When you don't eat enough the body assumes that it is starving and goes into emergency starvation mode. When the body is in starvation mode it stores every possible calorie as fat.

It stores fat so that if food is not available the body will have stored fat to use as fuel. So when you restrict calories you are actually forcing your body to make and store fat.

Why diets don't work

Starvation mode is the reason why people who diet don't lose weight, or lose weight and put it back on when the diet is over.

Dieting will not cause long-term fat loss. Only changing the way that you eat will do that.

If you want to lose fat you should be regularly giving your body the food that it needs to steadily burn calories.

Six meals a day

Nutrition experts agree that if you really want to lose fat and keep it off you should eat six small meals a day. Those meals should be mostly protein and some healthy carbs.

If you do that you will be shocked at how fast you will lose fat. Even that stubborn belly fat will fall off quickly if you are eating six small meals each day that are mostly protein.

The key is to keep the meals small. A couple of hard-boiled eggs and a protein bar might seem like a snack right now, but that would be a good meal if you are eating small meals.

You should be eating small amounts every 3-4 hours if you want burn fat fast.

Most people find it hard to imagine eating six meals a day, especially with a busy schedule of work and other commitments.

Here are some easy ways to change from three meals each day to six small meals:

- Pick a protein and one other food. You can't go wrong with this formula. A burger and some mashed cauliflower might be one meal. Some cheese and vegetables might be another. A third might be some yogurt and some nuts.

- Keep food with you. Once you start eating this way you will start to get hungry every few hours. Keep some string cheese, yogurt, fruit, or hard-boiled eggs with you so that you always have healthy food close at hand.

- Set an alarm. If you usually go the entire day without eating and find it hard to remember to eat set an alarm on your phone or tablet to remind you when it's time to eat. After a few weeks of this your body will naturally be hungry every few hours and that will be your reminder to eat.

- Write down what you eat. Keep a food journal to write down what meals you have already eaten. That will help you stay on schedule and make sure that you're eating mostly protein.

If you found these eating habits so far quite helpful, I would really appreciate it if you could take 30 seconds to leave me a positive review on my Amazon book page. Thank you!

Powerful Workout Habits

Exercise is essential for burning belly fat and for staying healthy.

Your body is made to move! Being active has a huge variety of health benefits including burning fat, building muscle, and keeping you healthy.

Exercise doesn't have to be a chore

Most people know that they should exercise more, but they think that exercise is boring and they don't want to do it. That's why they don't make physical activity a priority.

But exercise doesn't have to be dull, boring, or something that you have to force yourself to do.

Exercise can be so much fun that you won't even realize how many calories you are burning or how much fat you are burning.

Exercise for life

In order to burn fat, lose weight and keep it off you will have to change your attitude about exercise.

Exercise isn't something that you do just to lose a few pounds. A physically active lifestyle is the key to getting healthy now and staying healthy in the future.

If you live an active life you will lower your risk of heart disease, diabetes, and other serious health conditions that can be caused by a sedentary lifestyle and excess belly fat.

Stop making excuses

- I don't have time to work out.
- Exercise is boring.
- I don't like any kind of exercise.
- I don't have money for expensive gyms.
- My life is too hectic to work out regularly.

Do those excuses sound familiar to you?

Well it's time to stop making excuses and start being active. These powerful workout habits will show you that everyone can exercise no matter what their circumstances are.

Get up. Get active. Burn belly fat and lose weight. It really is that simple.

Workout Habit #1 – Set Fitness Goals

Setting fitness goals is an important part of becoming more active. When you set fitness goals you will know what you are working towards. Setting specific goals will also help you stay motivated to keep working out. Every time you make one of your fitness goals a reality you will want to keep going to reach another goal.

Set realistic goals

When you set fitness goals you should always choose goals that realistic for your circumstances. Working out every day might not be a realistic option for you because of your schedule or other obligations. But that doesn't mean you can't exercise.

Set a fitness goal to work out three times each week for an hour each time. That's a realistic goal that will help you get fit and lose belly fat.

If you choose goals that you're going to have a hard time meeting you might get discouraged and give up on working out altogether which would make it a lot harder to lose weight.

Share your goals

Let your friends and family know about the fitness goals that you set. There is a much better chance of success when you share your goals with other people.

When your family and friends are expecting you to work on your goals it's hard to tell them that you stopped working out or haven't worked out in a while. That can be good motivation to keep you on a regular work out schedule.

Keep track of your progress by writing down your workouts or sharing them on social media. You might even inspire some of your loved ones to start exercising.

Make an action plan

Once you decide what your fitness goals are you should make an action plan.

An action plan will keep you on track and give you a roadmap of steps to follow to make your goal a reality.

Here are some things that you should include in your action plan:

- How often you are going to work out. Schedule your workouts and write down how many times you want to work out each week and how long you want to work out. Writing it down will keep you focused on following through.

- What exercises you want to try. Make a list of any exercise that sounded fun to you. You might not like them all after you try them but working through the list will give you plenty of workout ideas.

- Keep a workout journal. Write down your fitness goals and your action plans in a notebook. Each day write down how much exercise you did and what exercise you did. Your workout journal will keep track of your progress and remind you what your fitness goals are.

Workout Habit #2 – Make Working Out A Priority

The only way that you are going to find the time to work out regularly is to make exercising a priority.

When you are juggling a lot of commitments it's very easy to skip exercising so that you can get other things done. But you need to make your health a priority.

Carrying a lot of belly fat can lead to health problems. If you don't make your own health a priority you could develop diabetes or other serious health conditions.

Exercise is important

Exercise does more than help you lose weight. Regular exercise builds strong muscles and keeps your body healthy.

Human bodies are made to be active. Sitting behind a desk all day is not healthy. The more you exercise the better you will feel. You need to get up and get moving at least once a day.

The mental benefits of exercise

The benefits of exercise aren't just physical. Working out is a fabulous way to manage stress and anxiety.

When you exercise your brain releases endorphins. Endorphins are what makes you feel great after you win something, or when you spend time with people that you love.

You can get that same feeling of joy and happiness from working out. And you can feel that way every day if you exercise every day.

Put yourself first

Sometimes it's ok to be selfish and put yourself first. This is one of those times.

Your health needs to be a priority and you need to take it seriously. Make time for exercise because you need it to feel better and look better.

Think you don't have time to exercise? You have more time than you realize.

Try some of these easy ways to make exercise a priority every day:

- Get up 30 minutes earlier. Go for a walk or do some yoga.

- Take a 10-minute walk on your break at work. Do that twice a day.

- Take a walk on your lunch break or go to the gym.

- Park your car in the back of the lot so that you have to walk further to get to and from work each day.

- Take the stairs.

- Walk around the entire store once before you get what you need and leave.

Workout Habit #3 – Get into a Workout Routine

Habits are hard to break. Once you make working out a habit you are more likely to do it every day.

It takes about two weeks for a new activity to become a habit. So, if you work out every day for two weeks you are much more likely to keep doing it.

Can you invest two weeks in your health? Yes, you can!

Two weeks of daily workouts is a small price to pay to burn fat and be healthy for life.

Find exercise that you enjoy

The key to establishing a good workout routine is to find an exercise that you really enjoy.

You can always add new and exciting things to your workouts to keep them interesting. But the workout that you do every day should be something that you really like to do or you won't want to do it every day.

The workout you choose for your daily workout doesn't have to be something that is very intense or high speed.

Taking a 30-minute walk every day is a great exercise routine. Or going for a bike ride every day.

Simple activities that you really enjoy will keep you coming back for more every day.

Workout at the same time every day

Another important part of establishing a workout routine is to exercise at the same time each day.

After two weeks of exercising at the same time each day you will automatically think of that time as workout time.

Working out in the morning is the best because you will have more energy and more willpower in the morning.

But if you don't have the time to fit in a workout in the morning then you can find a time in the evening to workout.

Taking a walk after work or taking a bike ride after dinner is a fun routine to get into that will burn fat and help eliminate stress.

No excuses

While you are working on getting into a workout routine you have to make exercising a priority. Don't put off your workouts to have coffee with a friend, work late, or for any other reason.

You need to work out during those weeks to set your routine.

Here are a few ways to make sure that you don't miss workouts during those important weeks:

- Make an appointment with yourself. Write down your workouts on your schedule and tell everyone you're busy during that time.

- Keep a second set of workout clothes in the car. If you are hitting the gym on the way home or at lunch keep a set of workout clothes in your locker and another set in a bag in your car. That way you can't use the excuse that you don't have any clean workout clothes to get out of a workout.

- Ask a friend to call you each morning. If you want to exercise in the morning but are having trouble getting up for your workout ask a friend or family member to call you early in the morning to be sure you are up and ready to workout.

- Create a workout calendar on paper. Electronics are great, but using a paper calendar is better. Print out a monthly calendar and hang it up near your desk. Every day draw a huge X through that day after you work out. Seeing those giant X's everyday will subconsciously make you want to work out so that you can continue the pattern.

Workout Habit #4 – Add Weights to Your Workout

When it comes to losing fat, most people assume that they have to do hours of cardio in order to shed fat, especially stubborn belly fat. But that's not true.

Cardio does burn calories and is important for losing weight. But adding weights to your workout can help you shed fat even faster. Studies show that weight training is a very effective exercise for fat loss.

Why weights are important

Working out with weights might not seem like much of a workout. But weights build muscle, which is very important when it comes to fat loss.

Your body burns calories all day long just doing normal things. When you have a lot of muscle your body burns more calories.

So, when you work out with weights and build muscle your body will burn more calories around the clock.

That leads to a lot more fat loss than just doing cardio exercise.

Adding weight training to your regular workout can increase your fat loss by as much 50%.

You don't need a lot of expensive equipment

Most people don't work out with weights because they think they would have to buy an expensive weight set that they don't know how to use.

But you don't have to buy expensive weights. You don't have to buy anything at all.

If you go to a gym you have access to weights. If you don't go to a gym and workout at home you can use your own bodyweight to perform weight-training exercises. You can burn fat and build muscle without having to buy a single weight.

There are plenty of exercises that you can do at home using your own bodyweight. And once you have mastered those exercises you may find that you want to invest in some weights and start a weight-training program.

But if you are on a tight budget you can start weight training without buying a single thing.

Here are some ways to get started on a weight-training program:

- Talk to a professional trainer. Most gyms have professional trainers on staff. If you don't belong to a gym you can usually get one free session with a personal trainer before you need to sign up. That one session can give you some great information about weight training.

- Look online. There are many forums and websites for people who want to start weight training. You can get advice and information from people who have been where you are and can recommend programs and equipment.

- Check out the library. Many popular exercise magazines and books can be found for free at the local library. Browse through them and make photocopies of any weight training programs that you want to try.

- Visit a sporting goods store. If you do want to invest in a set of weights to use at home visit a sporting goods store and talk to an associate. A trained associate can help you find the best set of beginner weights to buy for your fitness level.

Workout Habit #5 – Stay Hydrated

You already know that drinking water can help you lose weight. But did you know that you need to drink water when you're exercising too?

Don't just have a massive gulp of water after a workout, but consistently hydrate *during* the workout. Staying hydrated during a workout is very important.

If you get dehydrated while you are exercising you could develop muscle cramps that can ruin your workout and even cause injuries.

You also could become dizzy or light-headed if you are sweating a lot and not replacing all the fluid that you are losing through sweat.

What happens if you get dehydrated

If you get dehydrated during a period of intense physical activity the toxins that your body is releasing are not getting flushed out. That can lead to illness or other problems.

Also, your muscles can seize and cramp if you don't have enough water in your body during working out which can hurt a lot and bring your workout to a screeching halt.

Cramps and muscle spasms can also cause other injuries that can make it impossible to exercise for weeks.

When you can't exercise you won't be able to lose fat. So, drinking water while you work out is very important.

Water vs. sports drinks

Plain water is better for you during a workout than a sports drink.

Sports drinks contain a lot of carbs and a lot of sugar. The carbs in sports drinks aren't the healthy kind. They are the kind that ends up stored in your body as fat. So, drinking a sports drink while you are working out can actually cause you to gain fat instead of losing it.

If you want to make sure that your electrolytes are balanced you can add some orange or lemon juice to the water that you drink. Citrus fruit juice helps your body stay hydrated naturally.

Here are a few more tips for staying hydrated during a workout:

- Start drinking water before your workout. You know you will be losing fluid when you work out, so drinking water before you start working out will help you stay hydrated longer. About an hour before your workout start drinking water.

- Drink room temperature water during your workout. Drinking ice-cold water during a workout can lead to cramps. Make sure you have some room temperature water to drink during your exercise.

- Drink after your workout. Your body will continue burning calories for several hours after you are done working out. Keep drinking water throughout that time to make sure you stay hydrated.

- Keep water with you. Carry a water bottle with you that you can refill. You should also keep some bottled water in your car or in your desk so that you always have some with you.

Workout Habit #6 – Work on Your Core

Belly fat doesn't just look bad. It raises your risk of serious diseases like diabetes and heart disease.

Your core muscles are the muscles in your abdominal area, back and sides. Core workouts will strengthen and lengthen those muscles and burn fat.

No quick fix

There is no exercise that will cause you to lose fat in just one area. But when you regularly exercise your core you will lose inches in the core area.

Having a strong core will also improve your posture, balance, and stamina.

Pilates core workouts

Core workouts usually use interval training or weight training to work your core muscles.

One of the best core workouts is Pilates. Pilates is a series of stretches and targeted muscle building exercises that focuses on the core. Dancers and performers use Pilates to make their bodies strong and lean without adding a lot of bulk.

Pilates exercises were developed after WWII by a man named Joseph Pilates. He was a doctor who noticed that many of the men wounded in the war experienced a lot of muscle atrophy and weakness after being confined to bed with injuries.

He created a series of exercises that these men could do in bed in order to strengthen the core muscles of the body and keep them strong.

Today millions of people perform Pilates exercises to get six pack abs and to lose belly fat. Pilates exercises are easy to do and incredibly effective for getting rid of belly fat.

How to start pilates

Pilates workouts are short and can easily be done at home.

There are studios that offer Pilates classes if you prefer to go to a class. But you can also do Pilates at home using a DVD or watching a Pilates workout with instructions online.

All you need to do Pilates are:

- A mat. Any exercise or yoga mat will work for Pilates. If you have hard floors you might want to use a floor cushion or pillow under your mat.

- A strap. Pilates uses stretchy straps to help with stretching and to help hold the body in position during the exercises. You can buy inexpensive Pilates straps or you can even use a rolled-up towel or a belt to do the exercises.

- Water. Always stay hydrated during a workout even a workout like Pilates. Pilates workouts aren't very fast paced but you can work up a good sweat doing them. Keep water close by.

- DVD or Pilates book. If you are working out on your own you will need a Pilates DVD or book to demonstrate all the exercises. But that's all you need to get started! You can start burning belly fat with Pilates very quickly.

Workout Habit #7 – Use Kettlebells

One of the most effective workouts for losing belly fat is also one of the simplest. All you need to burn belly fat is a Kettlebell.

Kettlebells usually come in pairs but for this workout you just need one. They aren't expensive and you can find them at any sporting goods store.

25-50 Kettlebell swings per day can dramatically shape your core and get rid of belly fat.

What is a kettlebell swing?

A Kettlebell Swing is a move that comes from the popular Crossfit style of workout. Stand with your weight distributed evenly on both feet and your feet apart. Holding the Kettlebell with both hands, pick it up and raise it to chest level.

Then with a controlled motion swing the kettlebell down between your knees. When the Kettlebell is just behind your knees swing it back up to chest level. That is a complete Kettlebell swing.

50 kettlebell swings? really?

Really! It's not as difficult as it sounds. You should never do more than 10 Kettlebell swings at a time. So, you should do 5 sets of 10 Kettlebell Swings.

If you perform those sets throughout the day it doesn't seem like a lot at all.

Do a few when you get up. A few more before you leave for work. You can do some at work or on breaks. Then finish up at night after you get home.

Once you get into the habit of doing Kettlebell Swings all through the day you will feel like you're hardly working out. But you will definitely the fat disappearing from your belly.

Your back, legs and core muscles will get toned and strong too, which will burn more calories.

Here are some ways to make doing your daily Kettlebell Swings more fun:

- Challenge a friend. Enlist a friend or a few coworkers to start doing Kettlebell Swings with you. Throughout the day you can keep track of how many each of you has done. A friendly competition will keep you motivated to keep doing them.

- Create a great workout playlist. Music is a great motivator. Fill a playlist with songs that really get you moving. You will have fun listening to the music and doing Kettlebell Swings.

- Reward yourself. At the end of the week if you have done Kettlebell Swings every day of the week reward yourself with some workout clothes, a new

CD or DVD, or a trip to the movies. Just don't reward yourself with food!

Workout Habit #8 – Put Some Variety in Your Workout

It's good to have a workout routine that consists of one activity that you really like to do. But just doing one thing can sometimes get boring. It also can lead to a plateau in your weight loss.

Adding new activities and new intensity levels to your workout will keep it interesting. It will provide more of a challenge so that you will lose more fat.

Try new workouts

A great way to spice up your workout routine is to add a new activity a few times each week. You can try going to the gym instead of walking a couple of days each week. Or try swimming instead of biking on alternate days of the week.

When you try new things, you may find out that there are activities that you like better than what you're currently doing. At the very least you will get to try something new and burn some more calories.

Set a training goal

If you don't want to change the activity that you're doing you can try setting a new goal for yourself. If you like walking think about entering a 5K. If you like biking consider entering a race or possibly trying a triathlon.

Challenge yourself to achieve something big with your workouts.

Participate in charity events

There is a huge variety of fitness related charity events that are put on to raise money.

Consider signing up to raise money by getting friends and family to pledge money for every mile you walk or bike, every lap you swim, or every hour you spend doing Zumba.

Look up some of the charity events in your area and start training for one today. You can challenge yourself and raise some money for a great cause at the same time.

Here are a few other ways that you can add some variety to your normal workout:

- Use smartphone apps. There are many different kinds of smartphone apps that do everything from make you think you're biking through the Swiss Alps to training you to run and survive in a zombie apocalypse. Many are free or cost next to nothing so check out some apps that interest you.

- Relive your youth. Create a musical playlist from some of the best years of your life. Listen to the different playlists while you're working out to inspire you.

- Blog about your workouts. Take photos and videos during your workouts and blog about your experiences. Invest in a GoPro camera so that people online can see what you see as you work out.

Workout Habit #9 – Get Up from Your Desk

If you sit at a desk most of the day you are literally sitting your life away. New studies have confirmed what doctors have been saying for years – sitting too much is deadly.

Sitting at a desk for 8-10 hours each day and then sitting at a computer or on the couch at night is the leading cause of belly fat. It can also cause diabetes, heart disease, and even cancer. It puts you at a higher risk for strokes and heart attacks.

To put it simply – you need to get up.

Walk and work?

One innovative way to get your work done without sitting all day is to invest in a walking desk.

No, the desk doesn't walk. You do.

The desk is specially designed to fit over a treadmill. You can walk at normal speeds and the desk keeps your laptop, phone, and other materials steady so that they don't fall or move around.

So, you can walk all day long while still getting your work done. These desks can be a little pricey, but there are also DIY versions for people who are handy with tools.

If you're interested in another type of desk workout you can buy a mini-elliptical machine that fits under your desk.

You can pedal it with your feet, kind of like a bike, while you are sitting at your desk. These mini machines are easy to move around so that you can take it home with you too.

An exercise chair

Another option for working out at your desk is an exercise ball chair.

You have probably used an exercise ball to work on your abs at the gym.

An exercise ball chair is the same type of ball you've used before. It just has a small seat and a back attached to it so you can sit in it.

The exercise ball chair forces you to work your core in order to stay upright. You can work your abs and destroy belly fat all day long with an exercise ball chair.

If sitting on an exercise ball all day isn't going to work for you here are some more ways to get moving during the day:

- Take the stairs. Even if it's just one or two floors going up and down the stairs all day long will get your blood moving and keep you healthy.

- Get moving on your breaks. Take a quick walk. Or hit the gym on your lunch break when you have time to squeeze in a workout. Get some of your coworkers to workout with you.

- Get up every hour. This is important. Even if you just walk from one end of the office to the other it's important to get out of your chair and move around.

- Do some office yoga. There are yoga sequences that are designed for people to do in an office or cube that will increase your circulation and reverse the effects of sitting for hours.

- Keep walking shoes at your desk. When you are feeling tired, burned out, or like you're losing focus put on your walking shoes and walk around the block. Even a quick walk in the fresh air will clear your mind and get your heart pumping.

Workout Habit #10 – Have Fun Exercising

Stop thinking of exercising as a chore that must be done and have fun doing it. The more fun you have exercising the more likely you are to keep doing it.

That's how you will lose belly fat and develop healthy workout habits that will keep you healthy throughout your life.

Fun exercise?

There really is such a thing as fun exercise. You just have to find out what it is that you like to do.

Try new sports and activities to find out what exercise you really enjoy. If you used to participate in some sports as a child why not try joining a sports team or league now to see if you still enjoy that sport? Or if you always wanted to ride horses or take up running do it now!

There's no time like the present. Start going for weekend hikes to clear your head and get back to nature. Sign up for a yoga class. Or try a dance class. There are hundreds of new activities that you can try.

Join a gym

If you want to try some new exercises all in the same place consider joining a gym.

Gyms offer self-guided workouts, weights, fun classes, and even some sports leagues and swimming.

You will be able to find a new activity to do every night of the week. That is what will keep exercising fun.

Join as a family and you can participate in family sports together as a family activity. Many gyms offer discounts based on where you work. You also may qualify for a bonus from your company for joining a gym.

Exercise can be fun!

If you're still having trouble seeing exercise as anything but a chore, stop thinking of exercise as something that you have to do for a certain period of time or in a certain place.

Stop tracking calories burned or worrying about how many miles you logged. Go back to the basics.

Go do some of these activities that are still exercise, but will bring the fun back to your workouts:

- Take your kids ice-skating.
- Go for a moonlight walk with your spouse.
- Go to the beach and swim.
- Put on some music and dance around the house in your PJs.

- Take a bike ride on a sunny afternoon.

- Do some gardening.

- Hike in a local park.

- Walk around the city you live in and pretend you've never been there before.

- Join a hula-hooping circle at a local park.

- Take up belly dancing

Workout Habit #11 – Consult A Personal Trainer

A great way to be sure that you are making progress towards your fitness and fat loss goals is to meet with a personal trainer.

A personal trainer can give you the kind of guidance that you need to keep working towards the goals you set.

A personal trainer can also help you set new goals.

Troubleshooting problems

Sometimes even when you are eating right and working out your fat loss can just stop. That's called a plateau and it happens a lot, even to people who are working really hard to lose weight.

Sometimes you need to tweak your diet a little in order to start losing fat again. Other times you may need to start a more challenging workout routine in order to kick start your fat loss.

When you hit a plateau, a personal trainer can help you figure out how to start losing again.

Many personal trainers also have some education and experience with nutrition so a meeting with a personal trainer can help you adjust both your diet and your workout to help you get where you want to be.

Personal attention on a budget

It's actually cheaper than most people think to have a few sessions with a personal trainer.

If you belong to a gym check your membership agreement. Some gyms will include a few personal training sessions each month as part of your membership fee. Other gyms have resident personal trainers who don't charge a lot for private sessions.

If your gym has personal trainers who accept private clients you can just schedule a session or two if that's all you need. If you don't belong to a gym you can ask friends who do to recommend a personal trainer or you can find one online.

If the cost is more than you can afford, think about getting some friends together and splitting the cost. A group session with a personal trainer can still provide some great information and insights.

Here are some of the things that a personal trainer can do for you:

- Create a specific meal plan based on your activity level, lifestyle and income.

- Create a personalized workout plan to maximize fat loss.

- Provide coaching and mentoring.

- Weigh and measure you to keep track of your progress.

- Keep you motivated.

- Suggest new workouts that you can try if you're bored.

- Suggest supplements that can help you get past the plateau.

Workout Habit #12 – Keep Workout Gear with You

This habit is the one that will keep you in your fitness routine no matter what happens in your day-to-day life. In order to get a good workout in you need to have gear with you.

In fact, you should have multiple sets of gear with you.

No excuses

Investing in a few sets of workout clothes and workout shoes is a small price to pay for being able to eliminate your best excuse to workout.

If you have clothes and shoes always with you then you are always ready to exercise.

Whether you want to hit the gym at lunch or decide to join some coworkers for a run after work or want to go on a hike while you're visiting a friend for the weekend keeping gear with you means you have no excuse not to workout.

Multiple gym bags

If you are serious about losing belly fat and exercising more you really need four sets of gear and four bags.

Keep one bag always packed and by the door at home so you can grab it and go.

Keep another set in your car so that there are always workout clothes nearby.

The third set you should keep at the office in case you want to exercise on your breaks.

And the fourth set you should keep at the gym so that you always have a spare set ready in case you need one.

What you need in your gym bags

You should also be sure that you have all the things you will need to work out and clean up afterward in your gym bags. Being prepared will make it easy and convenient to fit exercise into your day.

Each bag should contain things like:

- Workout shoes
- Several pairs of clean socks
- Tee shirts
- A sweatshirt or jacket
- Bottled water
- A protein bar or two
- Baby wipes for cleaning up after a workout
- Soap and shampoo
- Deodorant
- Make up and a hairbrush
- A mirror or compact

Workout Habit #13 – Buy High Quality Workout Gear

If you're on a budget you might be tempted to skimp when it comes to workout clothes. After all, why pay a lot for clothes that you're going to sweat in, wad up in your gym bag, and probably not wash for weeks at a time?

But there are some very good reasons to pay a little more for workout gear.

Prevent injuries

One place you definitely shouldn't skimp on is the shoes you buy for working out. If you don't have the right support for your feet you can develop serious foot and leg problems.

Also, wearing shoes that don't support your feet make you more likely to trip, stumble, or fall. If you fall you could hurt yourself badly and make it impossible to exercise.

If you are on a tight budget there are ways that you can get high quality sneakers for less.

Shop during sales. Look for brand name shoes at closeout stores. Use coupons or discount deals. Look for online shopping codes that will give you a few dollars off.

Combining all of these "money-savers" means that you can get the quality you need at a good price.

Durability

Yes, those cheap shirts and shorts that you buy from the discount store might get you through workouts for a few weeks. But cheaper usually means lower quality. So those clothes won't last very long, especially if they are going through a lot of abuse.

Replacing them will cost more and it might interrupt your workout routine if you have to take the time to shop for more clothes.

Skip the hassles of dealing with cheap workout gear and invest in higher quality clothes. It is worth the cost.

If you really can't afford higher quality workout gear see if you can borrow some from friends or find some in a secondhand store. Often people who give up working out donate their brand name clothes to secondhand stores.

Performance

Once you start to take your workout seriously you'll appreciate the higher performance of good workout gear.

Having tops and jackets that wick sweat and keep you warm will help you perform better. Better quality pants and shorts will give your legs the support they need.

Here's a few more ways to save money on high quality athletic wear:

- Shop at outlet stores. Many brands have outlet stores where you can get closeouts for discounted prices.

- Get group deals. If you and your friends go in together and bulk order high performance clothes you can usually get a wholesale discount.

- Checkout sporting goods stores and secondhand equipment shops. Skip the pricey boutiques and look for clothes at the same stores where you are buying other workout gear. You can often get great deals there.

Workout Habit #14 – Exercise at Work

One of the best healthy habits is exercising at work. Sitting all day can cause a lot of health problems.

Getting a good workout in during the day can help offset the effects of sitting and working all day. Even if you don't want to hit the gym on your lunch break there are ways to get your workout in at work.

Walking

Walking is a great exercise. It helps circulation and it's a low impact way to get some exercise in. You don't want to worry about breaking a sweat or being too exhausted to continue working.

If you keep a set of workout clothes and walking shoes in your desk or in a gym bag in the corner of your office you can quickly change and go for a walk either on your breaks or on your lunch break.

Walking on your breaks can add up to a nice workout even though each break is short.

Aerobics

If walking isn't something that you enjoy you can start an aerobics program at work. See if some of your coworkers would be interested in participating in a Zumba session.

Or hire a Yoga instructor to come in and teach a Yoga class during lunch a few days each week. If everyone splits the cost it won't be expensive.

Working out together can be a great way to raise morale and lower company health costs. You may even get a discount on your health costs because you are taking steps to lose weight.

Here are some other fun ways to get in some extra exercise at work:

- Desk Yoga. There are plenty of programs on smartphone apps and on DVDs that will show you Yoga sequences you can do at your desk.

- Office games. When the weather is nice grab your coworkers on breaks or lunches and go outside to play kickball, volleyball or other games.

- Run the stairs. Who needs a stair stepper when you work on the 5th floor of the building? Put on some workout clothes and run the stairs on your breaks.

- Park and walk. Try parking your car in another lot and walking a few extra blocks to and from work. That will give you a great workout and a chance to enjoy being outside.

Workout Habit #15 – Track Your Progress

When you're trying to lose belly fat and become more fit it's important to keep track of your progress and your activity. You won't be able to measure how well you're doing unless you know what you are doing. Tracking your activity and your progress will help you figure out what you're doing right and what you're doing wrong.

Weigh ins

No one likes getting weighed, but getting on the scale regularly and taking your measurements regularly is the best way to measure how much fat you have lost. You will love seeing all those inches drop off from your healthy diet and workouts. It's great motivation to keep going.

Fitness progress

When you first started working out you may have only been able to walk around the block, but now you can walk several miles. That's the kind of fitness progress you should be tracking.

A good way to keep track of your fitness progress is to keep a workout journal. Each day write down in a small journal what workout you did. Write down how you felt and how much of the exercise you were able to do. Then you can look back through the journal and track your own progress.

Activity trackers

An easy way to keep track of your workouts and activity is use to a fitness tracker. There are tracking apps that you can put on your smartphone that will track the distance you walk every day, how many calories you burn, and how many calories you consume every day.

Many of them are free.

You can also buy a fitness tracker that can be worn on the wrist or the ankle. These trackers monitor how many steps you take each day and other factors that can keep you healthy.

Here are some other ways that you can keep track of your progress:

- Use a calendar. This is an old school method that works well for people who are visually oriented. You can use any wall calendar or print a calendar. Use a special color pen or highlighter to mark the calendar each day you get a full workout. You'll feel a real sense of accomplishment when those marks start to add up.

- Use your clothes. When you start working out pick a pair of pants or a skirt that is too tight. Only put that item of clothing on when you are weighing yourself. Over time you will notice those pants get looser as you lose belly fat.

Workout Habit #16 – Exercise with Friends

It's a proven fact that exercising with friends makes you more likely to exercise regularly.

Exercising with friends is a great way to make working out more fun. It also gives you a chance to hang out with friends even if you have a busy schedule.

Accountability

Your friends aren't going to let you skate by with a halfhearted workout. They also will definitely notice if you don't show up.

When your best friend is at your door for a run and you are still in bed she's not going to let you off the hook. She will get you out there running.

If you work out with friends they will keep you accountable for exercising and that is a powerful tool to have when it comes to developing a good workout routine.

Fun workouts

Working out with friends is a great motivator to find new and fun ways to exercise. You can try classes together, join a sports team together, or just rediscover things that you used to like to do together.

A bike ride with friends is a simple but satisfying workout that will make you feel like a kid again.

Each month let one of the people in your group pick a new activity for you all to try. You might discover that you are really good at rock climbing, or that your friend has a hidden talent for marathon running.

Group workouts

Group workouts can also make it cheaper to find new and interesting workouts. If everyone splits the cost of a new activity or chips in to pay an instructor then everyone can afford to try new things.

Here are a few fun group workouts you can try:

- Zumba
- Crossfit
- Yoga
- Pilates
- Belly dancing
- Hooping
- Spinning
- Salsa Dancing
- Horseback Riding
- Rock Climbing

Workout Habit #17 – Make Exercise a Family Activity

One of the best things that you can do for your kids and for yourself is to make exercise a family activity. Family hikes, playing sports as a family, even just playing games in the yard will have huge benefits for both you and your kids.

Teach a healthy lifestyle

Adults mimic the eating and exercise patterns they learned as a child. So, eating well and showing your kids the fun of exercising will help them be healthy as adults.

One of the most important things that you can do as a parent is teach your kids how to life a healthy lifestyle that includes a good diet and lots of exercise.

Have more family time

When you work and have a busy schedule it can be really hard to find time to spend together as a family.

Exercising as a family is a great way to spend quality time together playing, laughing and talking. There are so many activities that you can do as a family you'll never run out of fun options.

Here are just some of the fun things you can do as a family:

- Go camping
- Take bike rides
- Go to the park
- Try zip lining
- Go swimming
- Take a hike
- Play soccer
- Play baseball
- Play tennis
- Go on a mountain biking vacation

Workout Habit #18 – Stay Motivated

One of the hardest parts of getting into a good workout routine is just staying motivated to keep going.

Everyone starts off strong and wants to work out often to lose lots of weight. But as the weeks go by it's easy to lose the motivation to keep improving yourself. That's when you need to know how to motivate yourself to keep going.

Look better

You want to lose belly fat to look better as well as feel better. But shaming yourself isn't going to motivate you to workout harder or more often.

Instead of looking at photos of yourself when you're overweight and feeling bad, look at photos of people who look the way you want to look. That will keep you motivated to workout harder and accomplish your goal of looking great.

Feel better

Another reason to keep working out and lose belly fat is to feel better. When you're tempted to skip your workout because it's cold or too hot or you're too tired, think about how great you feel after you exercise.

Remind yourself that working out is the cure for every kind of bad day. This will get you back into the gym.

When you're losing motivation and feel like giving up, here are some ways to stay motivated to keep exercising:

- Put some great music that will get you moving.

- Stop thinking about how bad you feel and just get moving.

- Call a friend and ask them to work out with you.

- Try a new exercise.

- Skip your scheduled work out and do something active that you just enjoy doing like swimming or horseback riding.

- Buy some new workout clothes.

Workout Habit #19 – Challenge Yourself

The only way to improve when it comes to fitness is to keep challenging yourself.

You may compete against others when it comes to playing sports but ultimately you are your only completion. You should always be striving to be better and accomplish your goals.

Healthy challenges

Challenging yourself doesn't mean beating yourself up. It means always trying to reach the next level and accomplish just a little more.

If you start out walking a mile each day when you can comfortably walk a mile, challenge yourself to do to two miles.

If you are attending spinning class two nights each week challenge yourself to go three nights per week.

Keep reaching for that next goal.

Going beyond your goals

Developing healthy workout habits is about more than just losing weight, although you will lose weight.

When you use these healthy habits to live a healthy lifestyle you will stay fit and thin for life. You will have a better quality of life, and you will be able to have the life that you have always wanted.

Accomplishing your fitness goals and then setting new goals will help you get ahead in life as well as in fitness.

You may discover that you have talents and passions that you never knew you had. But challenging yourself to life a healthy lifestyle is the best thing you can do to give yourself the best life possible.

Here are some ways that you can challenge yourself to keep working out and keep losing weight:

- Become a fitness instructor. Find something you love to do and learn how to teach it to others.

- Become a coach. Coach a youth sports team and teach a passion for fitness to a new generation.

- Learn a new sport.

- Open a gym.

- Teach a class showing others how to get fit.

If you found these tips so far quite helpful, I would really appreciate it if you could take 30 seconds to leave me a positive review on my Amazon book page. Thank you!

Powerful Lifestyle Habits

Staying healthy requires more than just diet and exercise. Belly fat, in particular, can also result from hormonal imbalances, stress, and other factors.

So, in order to lose weight and prevent excess weight from attaching itself to your mid-section, you need to combine a healthy diet, exercise, and a healthy lifestyle.

What is a healthy lifestyle?

A healthy lifestyle refers to finding some balance in your life. You need to balance your career, family, and self. When you do that, or at least try to do that, you will reduce your stress levels and bring some balance to your hormones – especially those related to your stress levels.

Challenges to a healthy life

Modern life is hectic, stressful, and can make it hard to find that balance that you need in order to be healthy.

But if you work at finding that balance, you can achieve it. You just need to make having a healthy life a priority.

When you put your health, both physical and mental, at the top of your priority list, everything else will fall into place. You just have to believe that achieving a healthy life is worth giving up some things. And it is worth it.

Without your health and well-being, it doesn't matter what you achieve, you won't be happy.

A holistic approach to fat loss

Doctors are now admitting that it does take a holistic approach that combines physical, mental and emotional efforts to lose weight and keep it off.

When you develop these healthy lifestyle habits and use them with the healthy diet habits and healthy fitness habits that were already discussed you will be in the best shape of your life and happier than you've ever been.

Lifestyle Habit #1 – Sleep More

There is a real shortage of sleep these days. Thanks to smartphones, tablets and other gadgets, people are always connected to each other and to the Internet.

Numerous studies have shown that reading screens before bed can interrupt your sleep.

And people who can take their work anywhere, often never are off the clock. All of these factors lead to a serious sleep shortage.

You need more sleep

Sleep doesn't just prepare you for the next day.

When you are sleeping your brain cleans itself out. Your body resets itself and cleans out all the toxins that have built up. Your subconscious clears out the clutter so that your mind will be sharp and alert.

You need to get at least eight hours of sleep every night in order to be healthy. But most people are lucky if they get six hours.

The damage done

When you're not sleeping enough you can develop a huge range of problems, including weight gain.

Obesity, fatigue, irritability, depression, heart disease and other conditions can all be caused by not sleeping enough.

How to get more sleep

There are lots of things you can try to get more sleep, but you should use sleeping medications only as a last resort.

Instead of medications try these suggestions to get more sleep:

- Turn off your smartphone and computer at night.
- Meditate.
- Exercise regularly.
- Listen to soft music.
- Read a soothing book.
- Drink some hot tea or hot chocolate.

Lifestyle Habit #2 – Meditate

Meditation is a great tool for relaxation and stress reduction.

When you reduce your stress, you will reduce the chance of weight gain.

Lowering your stress levels can also help you naturally lose belly fat.

Meditating regularly will also help you sleep better.

Meditating is easy

Do you picture a serene person sitting on a mat in an empty room when you think of someone meditating? Most people do.

But really, you can meditate anywhere. You can even meditate at your desk or in the shower.

All you need is a quiet space. You don't even have to sit down if you don't want to.

What you need

All you really need to meditate is yourself. But some people like to use tools like incense, candles, music, or soothing lights to help them meditate.

It's up to you whether you want to use tools or not. But you don't need them.

You don't need a special room to meditate in either. You can meditate at your desk. You can meditate sitting outside on a bench or under a tree. You can meditate in your bedroom or in any other room of your house.

If you have the space to dedicate a room to meditation – it's fantastic - but it's not necessary.

Learn to meditate

There are a lot of smartphone apps available that will lead you through a guided meditation. These are great for people who are new to meditation.

Put on some headphones and let a meditation guide walk you through a restorative meditation.

Here are a few ways that you can learn to meditate:

- Visit a meditation center.
- Go on a meditation retreat.
- Take a meditation class.
- Read a meditation book.
- Watch meditation videos online.
- Use a meditation app.

Lifestyle Habit #3 - Keep A Journal

Keeping a journal isn't just for kids. Journaling is a valuable tool for getting rid of stress, dealing with problems, and living a healthier life.

A journal is a great place to write out all your frustrations and annoyances so that they don't build up and cause stress. A journal can also keep you focused on living a positive and healthy life.

Use your creative skills

Art journals are very popular for adults. You can use paint, photos, stamps and other supplies to create beautiful art journals that are therapeutic as well creative.

Many people find that making art journals is a great way to document their progress through life. They will often make an art journal for each significant event in their lives.

Art journals don't have to be professional quality art.

No one will see them but you, unless you choose to show them to someone. They are a way for you to express yourself with a combination of art and words.

Stream of consciousness journals

Stream of consciousness journals, or SOC journals, are also great for reducing stress and improving creativity.

SOC journals can be just plain notebooks or fancy books depending on what you prefer.

Either first thing in the morning, or late at night, sit down and write three full pages without stopping.

Write about anything and everything that comes into your head. This will help you reduce stress, focus more, and improve your creativity.

Here are some great journal prompts to get you started. Write about any of these topics in your journal:

- What is your favorite memory?

- What was your first pet's name? How did you choose that name?

- What do you think society will be like in 100 years?

- What do you think your great-great-great-great grandmother would think of the world today?

Lifestyle Habit #4 – Reduce Stress

Stress is one of the leading causes of belly fat. Stress can cause a huge range of health problems including things like heart disease, strokes, diabetes, belly fat and even heart attacks.

Stress can be deadly and most people have way too much of it.

No way to avoid it

Unfortunately, there really is no getting away from stress.

Life is stressful. Work, family commitments, friends, commuting and all the other demands on your time can cause a lot of stress.

And that stress can make you fat. But you can fight back.

Reducing stress

Luckily there are lots of ways to reduce stress.

You may not be able to do anything about your work hours or your long commute, but you can manage stress.

Eating a healthy diet and working out will help reduce stress, but there are other things you can do too.

Here are some ways that you manage the stress that you face everyday before it causes you to get sick or gain weight:

- Make Time for Hobbies. Hobbies are a great way to reduce stress. Try something you've always wanted to try like making jewelry or sailing toy boats.

- Laugh. Laughing is a great stress reliever. Go to some comedy shows. Listen to the comedians that make you laugh online or on CDs. Watch comedy show DVDs. Or just spend some time with your friends and family members.

- Listen to music. Music is very relaxing and can dramatically reduce stress. Learn to play an instrument that you've always wanted to play or just listen.

- Volunteer. There's no better way to remind yourself how much you have than to volunteer. Volunteering will help others and help reduce your stress.

Lifestyle Habit #5 – Disconnect

These days it's almost impossible to leave work at the office, disconnect from the Internet, and just focus on relaxing.

Everyone has a smartphone or a tablet and a computer.

After working on the computer all day, people come home and spend all night on their smartphones or tablets connecting to people on social media.

But there is such a thing as being too connected.

Not natural

You need a period of time to wind down at the end of the day and work through the stress of the day.

Instead of coming home and getting online, you should be working out, or spending time with family and friends, or spending time on your hobbies. It's not natural or healthy to be in front of a screen all the time.

The light from those screens isn't natural either.

In fact, the light from the screens can be causing you to gain weight.

When your eyes are exposed to the light from smartphone, tablet and computer screens that light tells your body it's daytime.

When your body thinks it's daytime it sends hormones through your body to wake you up and keep you alert. This can ruin your sleep.

Unplug for your health

The best thing you can do for yourself and your health is unplug at the end of the day.

Turn the smartphone off or put it in another room. Put the tablet away. Don't get on the computer. Give your body a chance to adjust and relax.

If you want to read then grab an actual book instead of an electronic reader.

Here are a few other ways you can disconnect and let your brain reset at the end of the day:

- Take a hot bath.
- Meet a friend for coffee.
- Write in your journal.
- Play with your kids.
- Go for a walk outside in the fresh air.

Lifestyle Habit #6 – Reach Out to Family and Friends

Spend less time on social media and more time in person with your family and friends if you want to reduce stress and be healthier. After all, social media might be handy, but it can't replace the experience of actually sitting with your friends and family members and talking or relaxing.

Real face time

Spending real face time with friends and family will help you relax, keep you grounded and focused, and keep you connected to the people that you love.

While using social media is a good way to stay in touch it will never replace family dinners, holiday celebrations, or picnics. Make time to actually spend time with the people you love.

Make the time

Everyone has schedules crammed with activities, school, work, and other commitments, so it can be tough to find time when you can all get together.

But it's important to make the time to see each other. Instead of spending an evening on the computer talking to your friends on Facebook join them for a drink at a local restaurant.

Instead of sending your mom an email to check on her drop by her house and have some coffee with her. Make the effort. It will vastly improve your life and theirs too. Here are some other ways you can make time to see your loved ones more often:

- Hold a family reunion.

- Offer to host a family holiday celebration.

- Take a family vacation.

- Take your kids to the town you grew up in and introduce them to your friends.

- Once a week meet your best friend for coffee or lunch.

Lifestyle Habit #7 – Be Active

You already know that you need to work out in order to be healthy and lose weight.

But living an active lifestyle is different from just working out. Being active in your everyday life means doing things for fun that will get you out of the house and get you moving.

Not just for the exercise but because they are fun to do.

The benefits of activity

Being active will do more than just help you lose belly fat. The more active you are the healthier your body will be.

Activity will improve mobility and keep you strong as you get older. Activity also will help you keep a positive mental state of mind that can keep you healthy and young.

Finding activities that you enjoy

Your workouts should help you find some activities that you enjoy, but not all activities need to be strenuous exercise.

Gentle activities that are fun will provide a lot of the same benefits as a workout like increasing your metabolism and burning fat. They will also help reduce stress, which will help you sleep better and prevent excess belly fat.

Here are some activities that you might want to try:

- Tai Chi
- Kundalini Yoga
- Water Aerobics
- Boating
- Hiking
- Gardening
- Dog walking at a local animal shelter

Lifestyle Habit #8 – Give Back

The happiest people in the world are the ones who give the most to others. A balanced life also includes service to others.

Volunteering will get you out of the house and can provide wonderful opportunities for you and your family.

Volunteering is the best way to remind yourself of everything you have instead of being focused on how hard your life is. No matter what your circumstances are you can find a few hours each week to volunteer.

A family activity

Volunteering is a great thing to do as a family, or you can do it by yourself if you want some time on your own.

Volunteering as a family teaches kids to be aware of the feelings and needs of other people. It also teaches them that everyone needs to help others out in order for a society to function well.

As a family, you can volunteer to prepare food at a soup kitchen, help out with the local church picnic, or help cheer up sick kids in the hospital.

If you want to volunteer by yourself there are plenty of ways to give back. Volunteers are always in high demand and short supply.

Not only is volunteering great for all these reasons, but there are many jobs that you can do, some of which will actually get you moving and increase your activity.

Consider volunteering for some of these organizations in order to help someone else have the chance at a better life:

- Animal shelters

- After-school programs

- Sports leagues

- Mentoring groups

- Reading to the elderly.

- Making blankets and other items for babies in the hospital.

- Helping with disaster relief.

- Building homes for the poor.

Lifestyle Habit #9 – Be Thankful

When was the last time you truly gave thanks for everything you have?

Being grateful for what you have is a habit that can bring you a lot of peace and joy. Being thankful is a mindset that successful people cultivate because it keeps them focused on the positive and not on the negative.

The more you give thanks for what you have the happier you will be.

Gratitude is for everyone

If you are not where you want to be in life you might thinking that you don't have that much to be grateful for. But that's exactly the kind of attitude that will keep you stuck in a negative cycle physically and mentally.

No matter what is going on in your life you have something to be grateful for. No matter how bad you think things are if you are alive you have a reason to give thanks.

Expressing gratitude

A great way to give thanks every day is to keep a gratitude journal. Your journal doesn't have to be fancy, although it can be if you want to decorate it.

At the end of the day sit down and list 10 things that you are grateful for in your life. Just writing down 10 things each day that you are thankful to have in your life can change your entire outlook.

When most people start to write a gratitude journal they think that they will never find 10 things every day to be grateful for. But once you start thinking about all the things that make you happy you will realize that you have far more than 10 things each day to be grateful for.

The main positives behind this habit in relation to losing weight is that it will not only help reduce stress, which leads to weight loss, but it will also keep you in a mentally happier and healthy state of mind.

Here are just a few things that you might want to give thanks for:

- Being alive
- Hot coffee in the morning
- A warm place to live
- Friends and family who love you
- Having good health

Lifestyle Habit #10 – Maintain Your Standard of Lifestyle

The last healthy lifestyle habit is to maintain having a healthy lifestyle by making it an expectation as a standard. Being focused on staying healthy and making the choices that you need to make in order to stay healthy.

This is the key not only to losing belly fat, but also to keeping it off and maintaining a healthy weight throughout your life.

Healthy diet

Now you know how to eat a healthy diet that will help you lose belly fat.

Choosing a healthy diet for years to come instead of dieting on and off will help you look great and feel great.

Remember that food is fuel for your body, not something you should be using to work through your emotions.

Exercise

You also know now why you need to exercise regularly. It's not just about losing weight. It's about keeping your body healthy and strong.

When your body is healthy and strong you will be happy and active for the rest of your life.

Living the lifestyle

In order to live a healthy lifestyle, you need to get enough sleep, make your health a priority, get out from the behind the computer and out of your house.

Give back, and spend time with the people that you love.

If you combine all of these habits you will be living the healthy lifestyle and you will have a healthy body and a healthy mind.

When you start to feel your life fall out of balance you can get your balance back again by:

- Focusing on choosing a healthy low carb diet.

- Working out more.

- Remembering to make your emotional and mental health priorities also.

I hope these habits were helpful for you, and if you feel like they could help improve your fitness, I would really appreciate it if you could take 30 seconds to leave me a positive review on my Amazon book page. Thank you!

Conclusion

There's a lot of information in this book to process. Take it slow and go through each habit carefully.

Try to implement one or two habits at a time and once you've got those down try a few more. Eventually you will find yourself with a balanced life and a lot less belly fat.

All the information that you need to lose that stubborn belly fat and get a more balanced life is right here.

You can come back to these tips over and over again if you need to remind yourself how to lose belly fat or if you just need some motivation to keep going.

Get started today to look and feel the way that you've always wanted to feel!

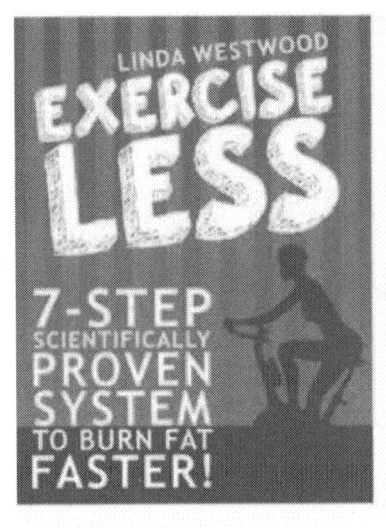

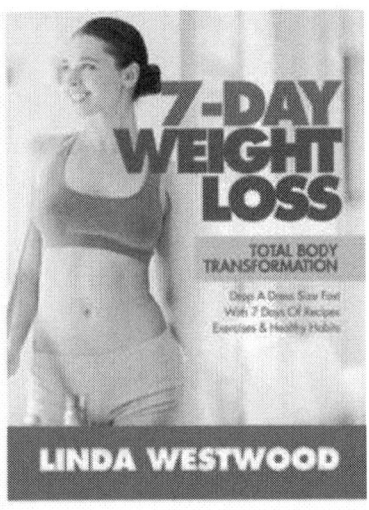

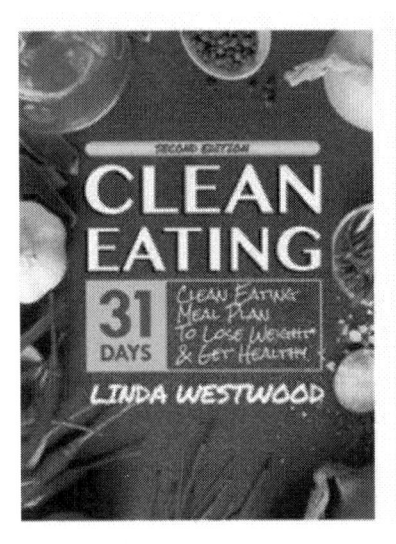

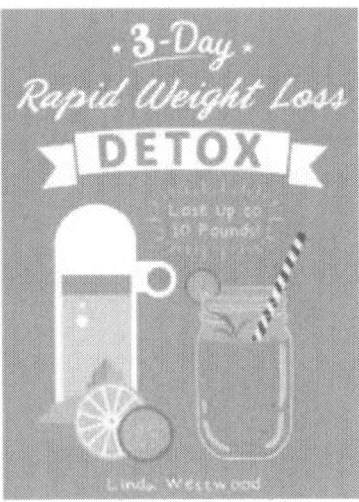

Check out Linda's books at:

TopFitnessAdvice.com/go/books

Final Words

I would like to thank you for purchasing my book and I hope I have been able to help you and educate you about something new.

If you have enjoyed this book and would like to share your positive thoughts, could you please take 30 seconds of your time to go back and give me a review on my Amazon book page!

I greatly appreciate seeing these reviews because it helps me share my hard work!

Again, thank you and I wish you all the best with your weight loss journey!

Disclaimer

This book and related sites provide wellness management information in an informative and educational manner only, with information that is general in nature and that is not specific to you, the reader. The contents of this site are intended to assist you and other readers in your personal wellness efforts. Consult your physician regarding the applicability of any information provided in our sites to you.

Nothing in this book should be construed as personal advices or diagnosis, and must not be used in this manner. The information provided about conditions is general in nature. This information does not cover all possible uses, actions, precautions, side-effects, or interactions of medicines, or medical procedures. The information in this site should not be considered as complete and does not cover all diseases, ailments, physical conditions, or their treatment.

You should **consult with your physician before beginning any exercise, weight loss, or healthcare program**. This book **should not** be used in place of a call or visit to a competent health-care professional. You should consult a health care professional before adopting any of the suggestions in this book or before drawing inferences from it.

Any decision regarding treatment and medication for your condition should be made with the advice and consultation of a qualified health care professional. If you have, or suspect you have, a health-care problem, then you should immediately contact a qualified health care professional for treatment.

No Warranties: The authors and publishers don't guarantee or warrant the quality, accuracy, completeness, timeliness, appropriateness or suitability of the information in this book, or of any product or services referenced by this site.

The information in this site is provided on an "as is" basis and the authors and publishers make no representations or warranties of any kind with respect to this information. This site may contain inaccuracies, typographical errors, or other errors.

Liability Disclaimer: The publishers, authors, and other parties involved in the creation, production, provision of information, or delivery of this site specifically disclaim any responsibility, and shall not be held liable for any damages, claims, injuries, losses, liabilities, costs, or obligations including any direct, indirect, special, incidental, or consequences damages (collectively known as "Damages") whatsoever and howsoever caused, arising out of, or in connection with the use or misuse of the site and the information contained within it, whether such Damages arise in contract, tort, negligence, equity, statute law, or by way of other legal theory.

Printed in Poland
by Amazon Fulfillment
Poland Sp. z o.o., Wrocław